Healing

Charles Frances Hunter

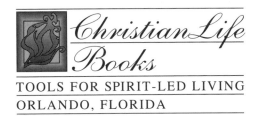

ChristianLife Books

TOOLS FOR SPIRIT-LED LIVING
ORLANDO, FLORIDA

CONTENTS

ONE

HEALING:
A LIFE-STYLE

Healing is simple, easy and uncomplicated because it is all done with God's power in the name of Jesus! Healing was a life-style for Jesus and for the early disciples, and it should be exactly the same today for every born-again, Spirit-filled Christian on earth.

However, since the time when the disciples lived on earth, only a few people — mostly ministers — have been gifted with what is called a healing ministry or gifts of healing. Only recently, primarily during this generation, have ordinary Christians discovered that they, too, can do what Jesus told all of us to do.

There is a big difference between the gifts of healing and being merely obedient to the commands Jesus gave us. The gifts of healing are still present in a number of Christians, but all Christians have a responsibility to obey everything Jesus told us to do. In Mark 16:18 He said that those who believe "will lay hands on the sick, and they will recover." This is a life-style Jesus was talking about, not a special gift, but a normal sign and wonder that would follow every believer to confirm the fact that they were telling the truth when they spoke about His miracle-working power.

Healing is not an end unto itself, but it is a God-given tool for us to use, just as Jesus and the disciples did, so that people will believe in Jesus Christ as their Savior and Lord and be born again. It is most certainly a tool which is vitally needed by Christians today. But even more important, it is probably the best tool we have been given to aid in the evangelization of souls. When individuals are healed by the power of God, it is extremely difficult for them not to believe in Jesus.

In the beginning of our ministry, success in healing was beyond our reach because we did not have the baptism with the Holy Spirit. Our church had taught against it, and we believed it was not for today.

Because of our intense hunger, however, God opened our spiritual eyes, and we received the baptism with the Holy Spirit in an exciting way. We never questioned its reality or the fact that it was a gift from God. We knew beyond all doubt that it was not just senseless jargon from the devil, as some have tried to teach.

Once we received this wonderful gift of God and spoke in tongues, we instantly knew we had received His power within us, and we believed that every person we touched would be healed — but they weren't! We laid hands on everyone we could. More results occurred, but it was nothing as we expected, so we went back to the Bible to see how Jesus healed the sick.

As fanatical as we were about wanting to learn how to heal the sick, we never lost sight of the purpose of healing: "Jesus' disciples saw him do many other miracles besides the ones told about in this book, but these are recorded *so that you will believe that he is the Messiah, the Son of God, and that believing in him you will have life*" (John 20:30-31, TLB, italics added). Jesus laid hands on the sick, and they recovered. Jesus commanded fever to leave, and it obeyed. Jesus spoke to diseases and evil spirits, and they left. But, strangely, Jesus never "prayed" for the sick. He healed them. Paul "healed" the sick, too (Acts 28:8). A light began to shine in our hearts, and a key of understanding opened a door of healing for us.

The principle of healing the sick was summed up by Jesus as: "The works that I do in My Father's name, they bear witness of Me. My Father who has given them to Me, is greater than all; and no one is able to snatch them out of My Father's hand" (John 10:25,29). "You shall receive power when the Holy Spirit has come upon you" (Acts 1:8a). "He who believes in Me; the works that I do he will do also; and greater works than these he will do" (John 14:12b). We are told in the Great Commission that all these miracles are to be done in the name of Jesus. Therefore, healing is simple because it's done with the power of God's Holy Spirit and by the authority that is vested in us when we use the name of Jesus.

Let's examine the way a doctor "heals" the sick. We will assume that we have caught a germ of some kind and have made an appointment to see our doctor. He examines us and gives us his diagnosis.

Then he prescribes a certain amount of penicillin or other medication and says, "That should cause you to get over this in two or three days."

You go home, and what happens? In two or three days you are well. What happened? Did the doctor heal you? No, he used his skill and knowledge and understanding to discover what was wrong, and he prescribed the proper medication for the problem.

What healed you then? The penicillin or other prescribed medication did.

Divine healing is similar in principle. The power is

injected by the laying on of hands for healing, but it is the power from the Giver of power who gets all the credit.

When we receive the baptism "with" or "in" the Holy Spirit, we have the most dynamic healing power of all within us. We are endued with God's Holy Spirit. When this divine power is dispensed into a sick body, the power does the healing. We always give glory to God and Christ Jesus. Always, when ministering healing, do it in the name of Jesus.

You Are a "Light Switch"

If you have ever turned a light switch on or off, you're smart enough to heal the sick!

Somewhere, not too far from where you are, is a generator (a power plant) that generates electricity. A wire brings this electricity, this power, from the source to your house and up to your electric bulb. The energy that flows from the power plant to the light bulb causes the filament of the bulb to illuminate. When this happens, we say the light is on.

Between the power plant and the light bulb is a switch or a breaker. The switch is designed to break the flow of the energy, the power, from its source to the destination in the light bulb. If you turn the switch on, the two ends of the wire are connected so the energy will flow through. If it is turned off, the wire is separated, and the energy cannot continue because of the gap between the power source and the light bulb.

In the same way the Holy Spirit in you is the generator or the power plant — the source of the power. Your hands are the on and off switch, and the person needing healing is the light bulb.

Now it is entirely up to you whether you turn the switch on or off. It is entirely your choice in healing to lay hands on the sick. Actually, the only choice you have is whether or not to be obedient to a command of Jesus. The power of God will do the healing, just as the electric current will light the bulb. If you want a dark room to light up, you can turn the light switch on. If you don't flip the switch, the room will stay dark. If you have an opportunity to minister healing to someone, it is the same kind of choice. You can lay hands on them and see them recover, or you can let them remain sick. If you have not yet received your generator, do so right now. Ask Jesus to baptize you with the Holy Spirit. Lift your hands up to God and begin to praise Him, but not in any language you know. Start expressing sounds of love so that the Holy Spirit can take whatever sounds you give Him and give you the language that will turn any ordinary individual into an extraordinary person! Let your spirit soar as it talks to God for the very first time (1 Cor. 14:2).

Be a light switch for Jesus, but be sure you are "turned on" for Him. Jesus said, "You are the light of the world" (Matt. 5:14). Let this be part of your being the light of the world.

Laying hands on the sick and healing them is one means that Jesus used to be the light of the world, to illuminate the way for the lost to find Him. He passed this earth-job on to us and gave us this healing virtue, this dynamic power, so we could effectively carry on all of His work while we are on earth.

(Charles)

8

TWO

LAYING ON
OF HANDS

P robably everybody who has a healing ministry has his or her own favorite way of healing the sick. Charles likes one way; I like another. My own favorite method is summed up in Mark 16:17-18 where Jesus says, "And these signs will follow those who believe: In My name they will cast out demons; they will speak with new tongues...They will lay hands on the sick, and they will recover." It seems to me that the simplest way to heal the sick is by the laying on of hands.

The Bible does not leave any doubt. It does not say *some* of you or just a *few* of you who believe. It simply says *all* those who believe are going to lay hands on the sick, and the sick *are* going to recover.

Believers are the ones who are qualified to heal the sick! But who is a believer? A believer is one who believes that Jesus is the divine Son of God and our Redeemer. A believer is also one who believes he or she can cast out devils; speak with new tongues; handle Satan and his demons; and lay hands on the sick and minister healing to them. We need to believe *all* the way if we want *all* of that Scripture portion to work!

You have to believe in divine healing if you want signs and wonders and miracles to follow your preaching of the Word. You have to believe that healing is for today, or else the sick won't recover when you lay hands on them.

You have to believe that you have been commissioned by the Lord Jesus Christ Himself to cast out devils, or you will never cast them out!

The greatest ministry Charles and I have is probably in the area of healing. We have never been afraid to step out and do the things God has called us to do. Sometimes we have experimented. The Bible lists many ways to heal the sick. But you can explore new avenues where God will open the door to effective healing.

But, you might say, it is not written in the Bible.

John said, "And there are also many other things that Jesus did, which if they were written one by one, I suppose that even the world itself could not contain the books that would be written" (John 21:25).

We must never depart from the *principles* of the Bible, but we can see many kinds of miracles that are not specifically described there. The occurrence of these miracles is not necessarily unscriptural. They may simply come under the authority of Scripture passages such as Mark 11:23 or Mark 16:18.

The first way Jesus healed during His earthly ministry was by touching people or by "laying on of hands." Touching still works today.

Sometimes people will say, "It is not God's will to heal." They do not know the Scriptures. "Jesus Christ is the same yesterday, today, and forever" (Heb. 13:8). If He healed yesterday, He will heal today. "Beloved, I wish above all things that you may prosper and be in health, even as your soul prospers" (3 John 2, KJV). A good verse to give them is Acts 10:38, where Peter told "how God anointed Jesus of Nazareth with the Holy Spirit and with power, who went about doing good and *healing all* who were oppressed by the devil, for God was with Him" (italics added). Matthew 9:35 says, "And Jesus went about all the cities and villages, teaching in their synagogues, preaching the gospel, and healing *every* sickness and *every* disease among the people." This is a wonderful proof that was sent to bring not only salvation but healing to His people.

It is God's will for His children to be healed. God anointed Jesus so that Jesus would have the power to do what God wanted Him to do. He thus put His stamp of approval on Him with the Holy Spirit and with power. Jesus said, "All authority has been given to me in heaven and on earth" (Matt. 28:18). It was given to Him — then He turned around and gave it to us. "Behold, I give you the authority to trample on serpents and scorpions, and over all the power of the enemy, and nothing shall by any means hurt you" (Luke 10:19).

Satan is the author of all that is evil, including sickness. God is not the One who sends sickness upon His children, but God can take sickness and make a miracle out of it. There was no sickness on earth until the devil appeared in the garden of Eden. His purpose in life is to "steal, and to kill, and to destroy" (John 10:10). He comes to steal your health, your happiness, your finances and your peace of mind.

I have heard people say, "God put this sickness on me to teach me a lesson!" I find that difficult to believe. Would God give something as horrible as sickness to His children? Would you do that to your children? Think how much more God loves us than we love our earthly children! "[And the Lord answered] Can a woman forget her nursing child, and not have compassion on the son of her womb? Surely they may forget, yet I will not forget you" (Is. 49:15).

God transformed sickness into a great miracle in my life after an automobile accident in 1964. I suffered a blow that caused me to lose the sight of my left eye. That could have been a horrible tragedy, but instead God transformed it into the greatest thing that ever happened to me. I found Jesus! After running from Jesus for forty-nine years, I finally accepted Him.

God did not cause that accident to happen. God did not cause me to lose the sight of that eye. But God used that circumstance to bring salvation to me, and He gave me my eyesight back as well.

There are many examples in the Gospel of Mark of how Jesus healed people. Read Mark and then read all of the other Gospels, searching for just one thing: *How did Jesus heal the sick?*

Mark 1:40-42 tells how Jesus simply "touched" the leper. He laid hands on him, and he was healed. Mark 5:35-40 says:

> While He was still speaking, some came from the ruler of the synagogue's house who said, "Your daughter is dead. Why trouble the Teacher any further?"
>
> As soon as Jesus heard the word that was spoken, He said to the ruler of the synagogue, "Do not be afraid; only believe." And He permitted no one to follow Him except Peter, James, and John the brother of James. Then He came to the house of the ruler of the synagogue, and saw a tumult and those who wept and wailed loudly. When He came in, He said to them, "Why make this commotion and weep? The child is not dead, but sleeping."
>
> And they laughed Him to scorn. But when He had put them all out, He took the father and the mother of the child, and those who

were with Him, and entered where the child was lying.

You will notice that He got the unbelievers out of the room. (Unbelief can stop healing from flowing.) The story continues:

> Then He took the child by the hand, and said to her, "Talitha cumi," which is translated, "Little girl, I say to you, arise." Immediately the girl arose and walked, for she was twelve years of age. And they were overcome with great amazement (Mark 5:41-42).

Jesus *touched* the little girl's hand. At the very moment Jesus *touched* her hand and spoke to her, life came back into her.

In this episode Jesus put two faith principles into action: He touched her, and He spoke. He issued a command to get up. Maybe if He had just touched her and had not said a word, she would not have gotten up off that bed. But Jesus issued a command. He said, "Get up," and she got up, even though she was dead. She didn't just lie there and say, "I'm dead. I can't do that!" She got up! When God touches us, we need to put our faith into action and do something we couldn't do before He touched our lives.

When I was hospitalized a few years ago, I was greeted at my bedside by the head nurse who said, "Eight years ago I was dying of Crohn's disease. I went to one of your services. All you did was lay hands on me and say, 'In Jesus' name,' and I was totally healed!" Then she added, "By the way, the little girl I had with me who had cerebral palsy was also totally healed when you laid hands on her."

It was probably a service where there were a lot of people, so we just said, "In the name of Jesus." When the Holy Spirit's power was released as we laid hands on her, she was healed by that same power. Glory! That was not prayer. That was not a command. That was healing through the laying on of hands!

We share these personal examples with you because we want you to believe, "Wow, I can do that, too!" Sometimes people will be in our services and say, "Charles and Frances can really go out and heal the sick. They just lay hands on them, and things happen!"

Charles and Frances Hunter *have no more power than you have!* But there *is* something that may be a little different about us. We *use* that power more often than most people do. We are two of the most persistent people in the world, simply because we do not get discouraged as a lot of people do.

You need to be persistent, too. If you lay hands on someone and nothing happens, try the next one. Lay hands on him or her. If nothing happens, don't give up. Sometimes Charles and I have ministered to the same person in as many as five different ways. We try commanding, laying on hands and casting out devils. Finally the persistence pays off, and we see the individual healed.

What if we were to say that it just wasn't a person's night, when he or she didn't get healed the first time? They might never be healed if we have that mind-set. But we continue in persevering to explore areas that are not fully described in the Word of God.

This is what God wants every believer to do: to step out in faith and lay hands on the sick and *believe* they are going to recover.

Do you know why I expect the sick to recover when I lay hands on them? Because I believe without a shadow of doubt that Jesus Christ lives His life in and through me. If I did not believe that, there would be no way people could get healed when I lay hands on them.

Throughout all of his epistles, Paul preached, "Christ

in you, the hope of glory" (Col. 1:27, italics added). Paul never portrayed Jesus as being outside a believer, dragging him along, saying, "Come on, I am going to make you lay hands on the sick. I am going to make you heal them!"

Because the Word of God says it, we have to believe that Jesus Christ is living in and through us. The knowledge that Jesus Christ is resident in my physical body is exciting to me.

When you fully realize that Jesus is living *inside* you, it will totally transform you. Then one day you will realize that when you put out your hand, it is the hand of Jesus Christ reaching out to heal.

Jesus said, "He who believes in Me, the works that I do he will do also; and greater works than these he will do, because I go to My Father" (John 14:12). So whom did Jesus leave on this earth to complete His work?

He left us who believe. He commissioned us to lay hands on the sick, using *His* authority. Remember — it's all done in the name of Jesus. It is in the name of Jesus that all miracles are accomplished, because Jesus lives in and through us.

Many times because of the size of an audience, Charles and I do not have the opportunity to minister to every individual in a meeting, so we say, "Every person, lay hands on yourself!" And it works!

(Frances)

Jesus' Command to Heal

One night a lady of about fifty years of age came to me for healing of her nose. She had broken it when she was four or five years old, and it had healed back at a crooked angle. I ran my finger softly down her nose. In front of my eyes the bone straightened instantly.

Months later we were having a Mexican dinner with a group of people, and I was telling this story. To demonstrate what I did, I ran my finger down the nose of the lady sitting next to me. Her mother, a minister's wife, was sitting across the table from her, and she remarked, "Look at your nose — it isn't crooked anymore!"

Faith had been brought to her by telling about a miracle, and the power went into her nose by the laying on of a finger. God did a twentieth-century miracle. Glory to His mighty name!

Have you noticed that the Bible doesn't say, "Lay hands on the heads of the sick and heal them?" Observe the healings we have mentioned, and you will see that hands were laid on a nose, on ears, on heads, on hands, on feet, on eyes. Because it is the flow of God's power that heals the sick, we get our hands as close as we can to the part of the body that needs healing. This allows the power to go directly into the sick part. Often the power goes in so strongly that if we touch a foot, the people will fall to the floor under the power of God.

Another suggestion is to stand as close as possible to the person being healed, because the power actually flows from all parts of your spirit, through all parts of your body, into the person near you. We believe that many are healed in an audience because the faith of believers causes the power of the Holy Spirit in them to become a force field that goes into those around them.

Jesus healed during His earthly ministry to bring people to believe in Him as the Messiah, the Savior (John 4:48). The disciples also healed the sick as a means of confirming the word they preached (Mark 16:20).

What a tremendous privilege, yet what an awesome responsibility.

What a trust our Lord Jesus has placed in us!

What a great commission He has given us — to be His body working here on earth, to do His good will. Jesus died not only to save the lost but to heal the sick

16

and free the captives from the evils of the devil.

Doing His will is so easy. Just simply lay your hands on the sick and believe that this dynamic power will go forth from the Holy Spirit in you into those who need His touch through you.

Jesus Himself set into motion this dynamic way of healing the sick. He wants us to use it to release hurting humanity and to bring them to believe in Him. Jesus said, "They will lay hands on the sick, and they will recover"(Mark 16:18). The Living Bible says, "And they [that's you and me] will be able to place their hands on the sick and heal them."

Jesus spoke this directly as part of His great commission. These were among His last recorded words while on earth.

Is there a difference in obedience now from then? Jesus has simply said, "Charles, go lay hands on the sick, and they will recover for you just as they did for Me. Frances, you go lay hands on the sick, and I'll heal them through you, too!" He has said the same thing to you, so there should be enough faith in each of us to obey Him.

The Word tells us that we Christians are the body of Jesus. If He did it in a body two thousand years ago, why should we try to change Him today?

It is an exciting thing to know that Jesus lives in and through us! And it is overwhelming to realize that the same power of the Holy Spirit is always available within us to do miracles.

If you haven't experienced the thrill of seeing God heal through your hands, why not try it?

Start right now!

(Charles)

THREE

THE
SPINE

It is estimated that close to 85 percent of adults have back and/or neck problems of some sort. Most of these problems are a result of some kind of injury. Usually the condition that occurs is a combination of misaligned vertebrae, muscle strain, ligament and tendon strain or tearing. The discs that sit between the vertebrae may also be damaged.

With such a high incidence of spinal problems, a large percentage of people need to be healed of back and/or neck problems. Charles and Frances have nicknamed ways of ministering healing to these injuries:

> The neck thing
> The pelvic thing
> Growing out arms
> Growing out legs

They call the combination of all of these "the total

thing." Therefore we will briefly review the spine and its problems.

The vertebrae are the bones that make up the spinal column. They sit one on top of the other. In between these vertebrae are the discs, or pads, that allow a certain amount of motion in bending and twisting the back and neck. All of these bones are held in place by sets of ligaments, tendons and muscles. In a person's back, the vertebral column is a channel made up of the circular rings of bone on the back of the vertebrae. This channel houses and protects the spinal cord, the main bundle of nerves running from the brain to all the parts of the body.

A severe fracture or dislocation can cause damage to the cord itself or to any of the thirty-one pairs of nerve roots that come out from between the individual vertebrae. Damage to a disc, which is the pad between the vertebrae, can cause it to bulge out and put pressure on a nerve root. This creates pain and, at times, weakness on either one side or both sides of the body.

Figure 1 at the end of this chapter describes which ailments are associated with disorders in each section of the spine.

The portion of the spine located under the base of the skull is called the cervical spine. This series is made up of the first seven vertebrae, the topmost being the atlas and the second one the axis. The head rotates from side to side on the atlas, and forward and backward on the axis.

The nerves from the cervical spine affect the face and the head, the neck, the shoulders and down the arms. Any pressure on these nerves will cause pain and interference with normal functioning in these areas. For healing in this area Charles and Frances do "the neck thing" (see chapter 4).

The thoracic (or dorsal) spine consists of the next twelve vertebrae, each of which has a pair of ribs coming off the sides, forming the rib cage. The nerves that come out from the spinal cord at this level affect the lower arms, the hands and the chest. For healing in this area they do what is called "growing out arms."

The lumbar spine consists of the bottom five vertebrae, where the nerves supplying the legs and feet come from between the vertebrae. For healing in this area they do what is called "growing out legs."

The next bone, rather larger than the vertebrae, is called the sacrum. It supplies support for the entire spinal column. The sacrum is also joined to the two hip, or iliac, bones (part of the pelvis) through a series of ligaments, tendons and the sacroiliac joints. Just below the sacrum is the coccyx bone, a short bone that comes close to the rectum, also known as the tail bone. For ministering healing to the entire pelvic area, Charles and Frances do what is called "the pelvic thing."

While ministering to someone with a neck or back injury, do not remove or readjust an orthopedic apparatus. To do so is illegal unless you are a licensed medical professional.

After the person has been ministered to, the Hunters suggest that you ask whether the pain is gone while the collar or brace is still in place. *He or she* may want to remove the apparatus to see what God has done. Let it be the individual's choice whether or not to do so.

Encourage the person to return to his or her doctor for evaluation, qualification or verification as appropriate.

(Roy J. LeRoy)

Roy J. LeRoy has been to almost all of our Healing Explosions. He is an outstanding chiropractor who practiced in his field for forty years before he retired. Now he shares his valuable knowledge and experience with the body of Christ.

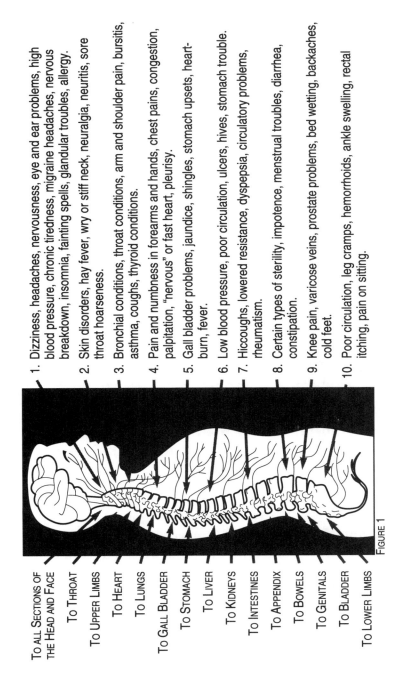

1. Dizziness, headaches, nervousness, eye and ear problems, high blood pressure, chronic tiredness, migraine headaches, nervous breakdown, insomnia, fainting spells, glandular troubles, allergy.

2. Skin disorders, hay fever, wry or stiff neck, neuralgia, neuritis, sore throat hoarseness.

3. Bronchial conditions, throat conditions, arm and shoulder pain, bursitis, asthma, coughs, thyroid conditions.

4. Pain and numbness in forearms and hands, chest pains, congestion, palpitation, "nervous" or fast heart, pleurisy.

5. Gall bladder problems, jaundice, shingles, stomach upsets, heartburn, fever.

6. Low blood pressure, poor circulation, ulcers, hives, stomach trouble.

7. Hiccoughs, lowered resistance, dyspepsia, circulatory problems, rheumatism.

8. Certain types of sterility, impotence, menstrual troubles, diarrhea, constipation.

9. Knee pain, varicose veins, prostate problems, bed wetting, backaches, cold feet.

10. Poor circulation, leg cramps, hemorrhoids, ankle swelling, rectal itching, pain on sitting.

TO ALL SECTIONS OF THE HEAD AND FACE

TO THROAT

TO UPPER LIMBS

TO HEART

TO LUNGS

TO GALL BLADDER

TO STOMACH

TO LIVER

TO KIDNEYS

TO INTESTINES

TO APPENDIX

TO BOWELS

TO GENITALS

TO BLADDER

TO LOWER LIMBS

FIGURE 1

21

FOUR

THE
NECK THING

We decided in the beginning of our ministry that God had made everything simple and therefore we should too. So we gave simple titles to all the things we do in healing to make them easy to identify and store away in your memory file. God enlightened us about "the neck thing" a long time ago.

We had a guest in our home who had a pain in his toe. I "grew out" his arms and legs, and the pain did not leave. So I asked the guest what the doctor said was causing the pain. I did this because we believe that if you don't get healed by divine power, you should see a doctor to find out what the problem is. Then we can know where and how to minister healing by God's power.

He said the chiropractor had told him that he had a thin disc in his back. Although the thin disc was in the lower back, the doctor "adjusted" the man's neck. This relieved the pain, but subsequently it returned.

In accordance with Mark 16 ("Those who believe...will lay hands on the sick," vv. 17-18), I put my two hands on his neck, placing my fingers on his upper spinal column. I did not realize where the other parts of my hands were actually resting. Later I discovered that the palms of my hands were on the carotid artery, the main artery on both sides of the neck that supplies blood to the brain. My palms were also on the nerves that go from the brain down the front of your body.

This hand position automatically makes your thumbs fall right on the temporomandibular joint, better known as TMJ. I was laying hands (thumbs) on one of the strongest muscles of the body. Was it accidental that God made our hands so that when we placed them in the right position we would be "laying hands" on three vital parts of the body at one time? Or did He plan it so that when we started probing into how to heal the sick the supernatural way, we would discover what He knew all along?

With my hands gently in place as described above, I then asked the man to turn his face slowly to the left and then to the right, then backward and forward. Then I asked him to rotate his head. At the same time I was doing what we later named "the neck thing": I commanded all the muscles, ligaments, tendons, nerves, discs and vertebrae to go into place, and the thin disc to be healed in the name of Jesus.

When he rotated his head, he shouted, "The pain is gone!"

We used this technique for years and discovered the results were phenomenal for headaches. Then one day Roy LeRoy told us what we were actually doing and why the results were so tremendous.

We have seen outstanding healings through the neck thing, not only in our ministry, but also through the hundreds of thousands who have learned this supernatural application of God's healing power through our healing seminars, healing explosions, video/audio tapes and books.

Almost 100 percent of neck problems; headaches; nerve deafness; arthritis in the neck; fractured vertebrae; deteriorated, herniated and disintegrated discs; and even broken necks and problems with TMJ have been healed by this application of God's healing power.

Large percentages of health problems will be healed through the basic healing application of the total thing, growing out arms and legs, the neck thing and the pelvic thing. This healing affects not only the spinal system but also internal parts, because nerves make muscles work properly.

(Charles)

The Sciatica or the Sciatic Nerve

Did you ever have a pain shoot down your entire leg, and you felt as if your leg was going to buckle under you? You were probably a victim of sciatica, a painful situation generally caused by a pinched nerve. But it can also be caused by a strained back.

This is one of the most painful of back problems, but one of the easiest to heal. Simply find the junction of the pelvic bone and the sacrum, lay two fingers on this area of the back (on the side where the problem is) and command sciatica to come out. Have the person bend over. No pain? Hallelujah!

Recently an administrator of a church came to me when the service was over and said, "I can hardly walk. This pain shoots down my leg to my toe, and it's killing me!" I placed my fingers on her sciatic nerve. Before I said a word, the power of God had healed her. Laughing, she said, "It's gone!"

(Frances)

FIVE

THE
PELVIC
THING

God will give you "witty inventions" and ideas beyond your ability and capability if you will be sensitive to the Holy Spirit and move when He moves.

At a service in Jacksonville, Florida, a man who was duck-footed, with his feet pointed outward, came forward. I certainly didn't know what to pray except to command his feet to turn inward instead of outward. But then a thought flashed through my mind. It seemed as if God was indicating it had something to do with the spine. I asked a chiropractor who was with us whether there could be a problem in the spine that could cause the man's feet to turn out.

The chiropractor replied that the man's pelvic bones were turned out and needed to be turned inward. In the natural realm, or even in the scope of chiropractic treatment, this would be difficult or impossible to do, but in God's kingdom and in the supernatural world it's no problem.

I placed my hands on the top of his pelvic bones and commanded the pelvis to rotate inward until his feet were normal. I was probably the most surprised person there when I noticed the entire pelvic area turn from side to side.

I wasn't doing it.

He wasn't doing it.

It had to be the power of God!

Just as quickly as the rotating had started, it stopped. The man fell under the power of God. When he stood up again, his feet were no longer turned outward; they were perfectly straight. Once again God had opened a natural-supernatural channel for us to learn more about healing.

It didn't take us long to figure out that if rotating in with the power of God would correct feet which turned out, then surely rotating out would correct feet that are pigeon-toed or turned inward. We tried it, and it worked. Since then we have seen many people healed of feet that turn in.

We've discussed this healing technique with many doctors on our doctors' panels. They've all agreed it could be invaluable in the healing of many other diseases as well. Because of the involvement of the entire pelvic area, many female problems are healed through the simple laying on of hands. Hundreds of women have been healed of premenstrual syndrome by the simple act of commanding the female organs to go into place and be healed while the pelvis is rotating.

Many problems in the lower lumbar area (the lower five vertebrae) and the sacrum are healed by commanding the vertebrae to be adjusted properly. Often a frozen or dislocated sacrum is restored to its right position by doing the pelvic thing.

Further, prostate problems often can be healed this way by commanding the prostate to become normal.

Colon problems are healed by commanding nerves controlling the colon to become normal. Any organ or part of the body which lies between the waistline and the hips often can be healed by this simple act.

It never hurts to look at a picture of the human body so you will know where certain parts are located. The pelvic bones are sometimes called the hip bones. They are the flat bones that make up your skeletal structure for the hip and pelvic area. If you will run your hands down your side in the area of your waist, you will discover that the top of the bones lie right in that area. That is where you place your fingers when you command healing.

Once you give a command in the name of Jesus, the pelvis will rotate or move in one direction or the other — if that portion of the body needs adjusting. If nothing is needed, nothing will happen, and the pelvis will not move.

If one side of the pelvis is higher than the other, command the high side to lower and the low side to come up. Don't underestimate the value of this simple healing process. The results are incredible.

(Frances)

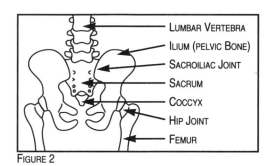

Lumbar Vertebra
Ilium (pelvic Bone)
Sacroiliac Joint
Sacrum
Coccyx
Hip Joint
Femur

Figure 2

The sacroiliac can assume many different positions. Sometimes the ilium (pelvic bone) rotates on the sacrum and causes one leg to appear short. Or it can go out of position, causing the spine to be crooked (scoliosis) even though the legs appear to be even. The sacrum can tilt forward and cause lordosis Q.24 (swayback), or backward and cause a straight "military" back. In all these examples, do the pelvic thing and command the sacrum to move into correct position.

28

SIX

GROWING OUT
ARMS AND LEGS
ISN'T REALLY GROWING
OUT ARMS AND LEGS!

You may have never seen an arm or a leg grow out. If not, you're in for a real treat. Watching the power of God move a part of the body is an exciting miracle to see. This is also perhaps the simplest and most commonly performed. It is a tremendous way to convince someone who is unsaved or not yet filled with the Spirit of the power of a living God who heals the sick.

You might want to try it on yourself. Stand up straight, put your feet together so that your toes are even and look straight ahead. Extend your arms in front of you with the palms facing each other, about a half-inch apart. Then push or stretch your arms straight out as far as you can. This exercise will help you test for spinal problems in the upper part of your back.

While your arms are stretched, bring your hands tightly together. Hold them together until you bend your elbows so that you can see the ends of your fingers. If you have a spine problem in the upper part of your back, the fingers on one arm will come out farther than the fingers on the other. If this is the case with you, then you have an opportunity to see a miracle. Stretch your arms out in front of you again, letting your hands touch each other lightly, but don't hold them tightly together.

You might want to say something like this, "Spine, in the name of Jesus, I command you to be healed. Muscles, nerves, ligaments and tendons, be adjusted in the name of Jesus." Using your knowledge of the problem, command healing as specifically as you can. Then give thanks to Jesus and believe it is done. Stand there for a few moments, and watch the miracle as the arm grows. You will see the short arm grow to the length of the other arm and maybe even feel the adjustment. The adjustment, however, will be either in the back or the neck, wherever the problem happens to be.

The instructions for growing out legs are similar. Explain to the person that while the back is being healed, the legs will appear to grow. Because of the way you will support the person's legs, you will want to watch your thumbs to see the power of God released.

The person to be healed should sit erect in a straight-back chair with his or her hips positioned tightly against the back of the chair. You should be standing in front of him or her. The person should extend the legs parallel to the floor without forcing the legs to stretch beyond the point of pain. Hold the person's ankles so that the inside tip of your thumbs is exactly on top of the peak of the inside ankle bones on both legs. Thumbs should be directly opposite each other and pointed straight at the floor. This allows you to help support the uplifted legs.

Remember the person's specific problem, and command the answer to the problem. Don't just command the leg to grow, but command the problem to be corrected, whether it be from an automobile accident, crushed discs, deterioration, scoliosis or whatever. Command it to be corrected in the name of Jesus. Watch the miracle happen!

This particular miracle has a peculiar effect on people. Because they can actually see it, it is usually remembered more than any other one. And because it is simple to do, you will probably see more of these kinds of healing than anything else you do. We could write several books on the back healings that have taken place in our services.

(Charles)

Two Healings at One Time

We've discovered something else about growing out arms and legs to heal back problems. Many times another needed miracle will take place at the same time!

For instance, a cowboy had three smashed discs in his back when he came to his first miracle service. By a word of knowledge I pointed him out in the balcony and said, "Your back has just been healed." Instantly he felt the warm power of the Holy Spirit move through his spine. His leg grew out, and he was totally healed. Up to that time he had been wearing a brace to ride, but he has not had to wear one since the night of his healing. However, another very interesting thing happened.

He was so wound up after the service that he couldn't go to sleep, so he picked up his Bible. He put on the glasses he had worn for thirty-one years and realized he couldn't see! Alarmed, he said, "God, You didn't heal my back just to let me go blind, did You?" He took the glasses off to clean them and discovered his vision was perfect *without* the glasses. God had healed his eyes at the same time that He had healed his back.

We didn't associate the two healings until God began

to show us a relationship between back healings and other healings. Could the back adjustment have relieved an optical nerve or adjusted an eye muscle to bring back the vision?

Another night a man who had been in an accident about thirty-seven years earlier came for healing. His back had been severely injured. Someone who was with him suggested that he also have his ear prayed for because he was completely deaf in that ear. Charles asked him what caused the deafness. He replied that it happened the same time his back was injured.

Normally Charles would have put his fingers in the person's ears and commanded the deaf spirit to come out. But before he could do that, God clearly spoke to him and said, "Grow out his leg, and he will hear!" Who has ever heard of growing out a leg to heal a deaf ear? We certainly had not, but Charles was obedient.

He said, "Sit down. God said to grow your leg out, and you will be able to hear." I'm glad the man didn't have time to think that over because he might have thought Charles was crazy. Charles measured his legs, and one was about three inches shorter than the other. He commanded the back to be healed. Then he commanded his muscles, nerves, ligaments and tendons to be adjusted and his leg to grow.

The leg grew quickly to full length, and Charles tested his ear. He could hear perfectly! He went all over the church telling everyone that he could hear with his deaf ear. He was so excited about hearing that he forgot to check his back for about an hour. Then he discovered his back was healed, too. Apparently the injury had pinched or damaged a nerve to his ear and caused nerve deafness. This was a new insight for us into God's healing world.

Hundreds have been healed this same way since we discovered there is obviously a connection between nerve deafness and back problems. When the tiny, hair-like nerves inside the ear have died because of a disease or high fever, however, we have learned to command a creative miracle of life to the nerves.

Because growing out arms and legs seems so commonplace, we overlooked the vast field of miracles that belongs in this type of healing. God has since revealed more and more miracles relating to back, muscle and nerve adjustments.

People who have had chronic back problems for, say, thirty years have been healed simply by commanding the vertebrae and discs to line up and be healed. So try it on everyone *you* know — you can't hurt them. We always say, "When in doubt, grow it out!"

On a recent trip to a foreign country, a person in a wheelchair had a broken spine. I grew the man's legs out, commanded a new spine in his body, and in less than thirty minutes we saw him walking across the stage, pushing his wife in the wheelchair he had been in for twenty years.

God is preparing the bride of Christ for His soon-coming return, and He will do it largely through the demonstration of His Spirit and His power. We want you to be a living part of this exciting move of God in these last days. Start growing out arms and legs!

Paul said, "And my speech and my preaching were not with persuasive words of human wisdom, but in demonstration of the Spirit and of power, that your faith should not be in the wisdom of men but in the power of God" (1 Cor. 2:4-5).

(Frances)

SEVEN

LEARNING
NEW THINGS

Ministering healing is a constantly changing and improving opportunity. The more we minister healing, the more new ways we learn. We listen to medical doctors and chiropractors and have discovered innumerable successful ways to help people.

Carpal Tunnel Syndrome

Recently a chiropractor told us about a common problem today among people who use their wrists a lot. Called carpal tunnel syndrome, it can cause such pain in the hand and wrist area that some individuals are unable to sleep or perform their work.

In the hinge of the wrist there exists a "tunnel" that houses ligaments and tendons. When the tunnel becomes inflamed or swollen, the passage is closed to varying degrees. Pain, weakness or other discomforts in the wrist area arise.

To heal carpal tunnel syndrome, place your thumb on one side of the soft spot in the wrist joint and a finger on the opposite side. Command the tunnel to open, both the inflammation and the swelling to be healed, and the tendons and ligaments to go back to normal length and position. Command them to be healed in the name of Jesus. There is a simple way to test for healing of carpal tunnel syndrome. Have the person put his or her thumb and little finger together to form an "o." Then put your forefinger in the circle and force the fingers apart. If the person has carpal tunnel syndrome, you can pull your finger through easily. Once it is healed, you won't be able to break through the thumb and little finger.

Miracles for carpal tunnel syndrome happen regularly. Recently Frances had her hair done at a beauty parlor in preparation for having our pictures taken. Her hair stylist worked carefully, feverishly and patiently to accomplish a perfect hairdo.

I noticed she wore a steel brace on her left wrist, extending about eight inches up her arm. When I asked her if she had carpal tunnel syndrome, she answered yes. She added that she had set sixty-two wigs that day. Because of the strain this had put on her left hand, she could hardly move her wrist.

I asked her if she would like for God to heal it. The minute she got a break I did what we had learned and gave the commands. We had tested the woman's strength, and there was no resistance when I moved my finger through the loop she had made by holding her thumb and little finger in position. After we gave the commands, we immediately tested her strength again. She was utterly amazed. She shook her wrist and in a few minutes had removed the brace. She was working free of pain. When we talked to her about two weeks later, she was exuberant with praise to God for completing this much-needed miracle.

A medical doctor recently called Frances to tell her

his excitement about divine healing success after he watched our fourteen-hour video series and read the book *How to Heal the Sick.* She told him about carpal tunnel syndrome healings, explained to him how to test this before and after ministering, and how to do it. About two weeks later this same physician called her again, but with even more excitement. He said many patients with carpal tunnel syndrome had come to him. Every single one was healed when he did what God had shown us. Then he asked with a laugh, "What should I do with the thousands of fliers I bought, telling how surgery could help heal the problem?"

A corresponding soft spot is located in the ankle area. For certain feet problems, the pain can be alleviated by giving the same commands. Simply hold your ankle the same way you hold your wrist. At the same time, command the twenty-six bones in each foot to go into perfect position. A third ailment, tendinitis, is healed by the same process. If you will be alert to the nudgings of the Holy Spirit, you will discover many new ways to see someone healed.

Tic Douloureux (Trigeminal Neuralgia)

Recently we visited with Hilton Sutton, president of Missions to America and a great Bible prophecy teacher. He shared with us for the first time that he had a problem called tic douloureux, or trigeminal neuralgia. We had seen few people healed of this painful affliction and did not know of any medical procedure that would help the problem.

The *American Medical Association Family Medical Guide*, published by Random House (New York, 1991), describes this affliction as pain from a damaged nerve. This kind of neuralgia rarely affects anyone under fifty except in cases of multiple sclerosis. The trigeminal nerve is a major nerve in the face. If it is damaged, the result is severe pain that is usually felt on only one side of the face. Although it is not life-threatening, trigeminal neuralgia can be distressing and disabling. We have talked to people who say it is one of the most painful afflictions there is. In fact, it is sometimes called the suicide disease. This same medical guide reports that the pain of trigeminal neuralgia shoots through one side of the face along the length of the nerve. It may last for a few seconds or as long as a minute or more. While it lasts it can be excruciating. Sometimes attacks occur every few minutes for several days or weeks for no apparent reason. They may then fade, but stabbing pains usually return with decreasing intervals between them. Attacks may eventually become almost continuous. In some cases occasional muscular spasms accompany the pain and cause a facial tic (twitching).

Hilton told us that for eight long and painful years he had suffered with tic douloureux. It was getting so bad that he was considering canceling some of his speaking engagements. Then he said, "The medical world has discovered a surgery that can stop this excruciating pain." We listened intently, because when a cause and a cure are discovered, we often find clues to a healing that God has in store for us.

He explained the type of surgery they perform. They drill a hole through the skull and go into a place where a blood vessel or artery is too close to a nerve. Then they place a medical wedge between the two, which stops the pain.

Our response was "Thank You, Jesus!" Immediately we laid hands on Hilton's head and commanded a divine wedge to separate the vessel or artery and the nerve. We gave thanks to Jesus. When Hilton called a month later, he said the only pain he had experienced since that day was a headache resulting from a stressful situation.

Another month went by, and we talked again on the day we were writing this story. Hilton said he has had no more pain. Glory to God for healing him!

And thank You, Jesus, for showing us how to heal tic douloureux.

Drug Addiction

A man named Al came to one of our services recently and told us an unusual story. Around midnight he was sound asleep in a motel room. The manager, thinking the room was vacant, entered the room. Al thought he was a burglar, jumped out of bed and, in his hurry, caught his feet in the bedding. He fell against a chest of drawers and hit the wall. This caused some discs and vertebrae to go out of alignment because they were fractured. The doctors said he had multiple fractures. Further, his muscles, nerves, tendons and ligaments were all torn badly.

For six years he had surgery every year, trying to eliminate enough of the pain so that he could bear it. To help the situation, the doctor had prescribed a strong pain killer. Not only did the excruciating pain persist, but the man discovered after a while that he was hooked on the prescribed drugs.

We sat the man on a chair and measured his legs. They were approximately two inches off. Thus, we commanded a creative miracle and the healing of all the vertebrae, discs, muscles, tendons, ligaments and nerves. We also commanded all of the scar tissue to be healed and then rebuked the pain in Jesus' name.

When he got up from the chair after seeing his legs "grow" out, he bent over and moved around vigorously. Then he asked, "May I run around the church?" He jumped off the stage, ran around the church, jumped back on the stage and then jumped up and down as hard as he could, shouting, "The pain is gone! I've been healed!"

Later that night we were ministering to people individually. Suddenly I saw Al again. God impressed me to go directly to him and pray the following: "Father, in Jesus' name, I command a new blood system, cleansed of all drugs. Thank You, Jesus. We believe it's done!"

We never recommend that people stop taking their medicine without the advice of their physician. But later Al reported to us that he threw all of his medicine away on the way home that night. He said he has never had one withdrawal symptom or been in need of the medicine since. In our communication with Al, we've found out that he has had no back problems. He's also been freed of drug addiction.

Do you see what we learned? A new blood system can correct drug, cigarette or alcohol problems. Now we pray for a new blood system for all addicts so that there will be no craving for the drugs, cigarettes or alcohol.

(Charles)

EIGHT

THE
IMMUNE
SYSTEM

You will be used in many healings because you know to what part of the body you should direct God's power in Jesus' name. To minister effectively, you will also need to understand the importance of a healthy, active immune system.

The following is a quote from the *Complete Home Medical Guide* (Columbia University College of Physicians and Surgeons, Crown Publishers Inc., New York).

> To understand allergies, one must first understand the immune system, whose misdirected response causes allergic reactions. The job of the immune system is to search for, recognize, and destroy germs and other dangerous invaders of the body, known as antigens. It does this by producing antibodies or special molecules to match and counteract each antigen.
>
> The key soldiers of the immune system are

the lymphocytes, the white blood cells manufactured by the millions in the bone marrow. The lymphocytes produce antibodies specific to each unwanted antigen. Circulating in the bloodstream, the antibodies attack the antigen, or protect the body's cells from invasion by the antigen, or make the invader palatable to roaming scavenger cells called macrophages. Antibody-producing lymphocytes or plasma cells are called B cells. When lymphocytes are activated, some of them become "memory" cells. Then the next time a person encounters that same antigen which earlier turned the lymphocytes on, the immune system "remembers" it and is primed to destroy it immediately. This is acquired immunity.

Apparently the immune system ignores cancer cells until they spread cancer. This may also be true of AIDS or other mysterious diseases for which science has found no cure. But doctors and scientists believe they may have discovered a way to develop an immunity to cancer cells.

We are planning to test a new area of commands for cancer patients, saying, "In Jesus' name, we command the memory of the immune system to be healed, so that it recognizes and destroys the invading cancer cells."

Many cancer patients have been healed as we bind Satan in Jesus' name by the power of the Holy Spirit, commanding the spirit of cancer to leave and the seed and root of every cancer cell to die. Then, by faith, we believe God for new immune and blood systems.

(Charles)

NINE

SEVEN STEPS TO MINISTERING HEALING

Jesus said: "Go into all the world and preach the gospel to every creature. He who believes and is baptized will be saved; but he who does not believe will be condemned" (Mark 6:15-16).

Step 1: Believe What the Word of God Says

And these signs will follow those who believe: In My name they will cast out demons; they will speak with new tongues; they will take up serpents; and if they drink anything deadly, it will by no means hurt them; they will lay hands on the sick, and they will recover (Mark 16:17-18).

I repeat these last eleven words: "They will lay hands on the sick, and they will recover." It is imperative that we believe with all our hearts that His desire is for believers to lay hands on the sick *with results.*

We must also believe Philippians 2:9-11: "Therefore God also has highly exalted Him and given Him the name which is above every name, that at the name of Jesus every knee should bow, of those in heaven, and of those on earth, and of those under the earth, and that every tongue should confess that Jesus Christ is Lord, to the glory of God the Father."

The name of Jesus is above the name of every disease that exists or which will ever exist. It is above the name of cancer, arthritis, cerebral palsy and Parkinson's disease.

Sometimes when we're first obedient to Jesus and lay hands on the sick, we approach the power that is in the name of Jesus, asking, "In the name of Jesus?" Instead we should approach healing with absolute confidence in the power that is in that very special name.

I made a very interesting typographical mistake when I typed the original notes for this book. I discovered that I had made a very interesting typographical mistake. I had planned to type "meditate in the Bible"; instead I had typed "medicate in the Bible." I laughed as I started to correct the error. But the more I thought about it, the more I realized that the Bible is medicine to our minds, bodies, souls and spirits. The more you *medicate* on the Word, the more you will be convinced that God heals today.

Nothing will keep us as strong as God's Word, and nothing will help in healing more than the Word. When you "medicate" on the Word of God, it will heal you of any unbelief. To be successful in the healing ministry, you must get rid of unbelief — the devil constantly tries to put questions about healing in your mind. But it is amazing to see what happens when you give the Word to someone to whom you are ministering healing.

I remember the day I was healed of diabetes. Not realizing that God had healed me, I was still taking my insulin and went into insulin shock in the Atlanta airport. As I fell over in the chair, my Bible opened to Psalm 30:2, which says, "O Lord my God, I cried out to You, and You healed me."

I repeated that verse until it became a reality in my mind and life. The same doctor who had diagnosed my diabetes two weeks earlier re-examined me and said, "You have a new pancreas, so throw away your medicine!"

I knew right then and there that I had been totally healed of diabetes. I haven't had a problem or sign of diabetes from that day to this. I believe that what God does, He does well. "He hath done all things well" (Mark 7:37, KJV).

There's power in God's Word. That Scripture passage in the airport gave me something to cling to. It let me know beyond any shadow of doubt that I was healed.

In 1988 I was healed of endocarditis (the inflammation of the lining of the heart and its valves). At that time God gave me another verse. The doctors had told me I wasn't going to live because my blood system was pulling off pieces of my heart. They said that when enough heart tissue had been destroyed, my life would end. The night after Charles prayed for me, a supernatural event took place right in our bedroom.

Although in my spirit I did not receive the diagnosis the doctors had given me, Charles took me to a heart specialist in Houston who ordered additional tests. When we returned home, I was exhausted and fell into a sound sleep.

I was awakened in the middle of the night and felt as if I had been hit on the head and chest by a two-by-four piece of wood. While I do not know if it was a vision or a dream, it was one of the most real things I have ever experienced in my entire life!

I looked, and there, completely covering my chest, appeared to be a huge, wooden book. On it was one single verse of Scripture:

Those who wait on the Lord
Shall renew their strength;
They shall mount up with wings like eagles,
They shall run and not be weary,
They shall walk and not faint (Is. 40:31).

Instantly, in that split second of time when God gave me that verse, I knew *that I knew that I knew* that I had been healed, because God had renewed my strength!

Many Scripture passages will give you confidence if you will remember them when you are laying hands on the sick. They are also beneficial to you in the event you yourself should ever need healing.

• *Hebrews 4:12* — For the word of God is living and powerful, and sharper than any two-edged sword, piercing even to the division of soul and spirit, and of joints and marrow, and is a discerner of the thoughts and intents of the heart."

We need not fear disease, because the Word of God is so sharp that it can cut through any disease or crippling situation in which we might find ourselves.

• *Isaiah 55:11* — So shall My word be that goes forth from My mouth; it shall not return to Me void, but it shall accomplish what I please, and it shall prosper in the thing for which I sent it."

• *Luke 11:28* — Blessed are those who hear the word of God and keep it!" Not only do we need to hear it, but we also need to keep it. You can be blessed just by hearing it, but you can be more than doubly blessed by hearing it and keeping it!

• *Mark 13:31* — Heaven and earth will pass away, but My words will by no means pass away." What a powerful comfort to know that His word will never pass away. You can rest assured that this is a fact which will never change.

• Romans 10:17 — So then faith comes by hearing, and hearing by the word of God." At times this is the written Word of God, but often it's the rhema word that God speaks into your heart. You know that you have heard from God when He gives you that special word, and that it will come to pass in your life.

• *Psalm 119:11* — Your word I have hidden in my heart, that I might not sin against You." When that old nature comes up in us, giving us an urge to sin, we need to remember, "Your word I have hidden in my heart, that I might not sin against You." It is amazing how fast the remembrance of that verse will keep us from crossing over the line into sin again!

• *Luke 4:4* — It is written, 'Man shall not live by bread alone, but by every word of God.' " *Every*, not just part, but by *every* word of God.

Step 2: Make Healing a Life-Style

Catch a vision of what God has called you to do. Then go out and do it. It goes beyond putting on a hat on Sunday mornings, going to church and, when the service is over, thinking, "Well, I did my *little thing* for the week, so here I go!" Then you go out the door and live just as you did previously, coming back the following Sunday, thinking that you're living the Christian life-style.

Real Christianity is a life-style that you live every moment of every day. There's no time off, no vacation time, because it's a twenty-four-hour-a-day thing, every day of the year.

I got saved at the ripe old age of forty-nine, and I went up like a rocket. I left the church that morning and tried to beat Jesus into the head of every person I met. I went up and down U.S. Highway 1, in Kendall, Florida, like a wild woman. And I was — I was wild about Jesus!

When I went to church the next Sunday, I was excited because of all the wonderful things that had happened during my first week as a Christian. I started out the first day to make Christianity a life-style. I shocked many of the "old" saints in the church who promptly said: "She'll never make it; she'll fizzle out. She won't last long. Those who go up like that come down real fast, and then they crash."

It's been more than twenty-seven years, and I'm still going strong, and I intend to keep on going stronger until Jesus returns. Peculiarly, many of those "saints" have backslidden since then. It has caused me to wonder about something.

What makes a person hang in there with God? What makes a person fizzle out? What makes a person hang in there with healing? Many times at a healing explosion we see people get so excited that they want to lay hands on everyone in sight. You see them laying hands on the sick in the hotel elevators. You see them growing out waiters' and waitresses' arms. But the important thing is not what they do at a healing explosion, but what they will do to keep from fizzling out once the healing explosion is over.

Charles and I have made healing a life-style. Everywhere we go we lay hands on the sick. We talk about Jesus and healing; we don't talk about anything else. We don't feel anything else is worth talking about.

The other night in a cafeteria a man came up to us and asked if we minded the interruption. After we assured him that we did not, he said, "Fifteen years ago you laid hands on me for deliverance from cigarettes. Although I haven't seen you from that day to this, I've never smoked another cigarette since."

What a whoop-and-holler time we had right there in the cafeteria. To me that is exciting news — and I'm sure there wasn't another conversation in the cafeteria nearly as exciting as ours. We praised the Lord right there in public because it is a life-style with us. It's not something that we pretend to have in the pulpit. It's

something we do every waking moment of our day.
The excitement of our first week of salvation needs to be part of our walk with Jesus right now. We should all notice the needs of others — whether we are in a grocery store, at work or in the church. Those people need you and me to help them find the answer to life.

The day I got saved I made a *decision*, a quality decision, and nothing could ever make me change my mind. I made an *everlasting* decision.

We must not vacillate. We need to get into the Bible, our holding power, instead of saying, "I don't think this 'stuff' works!" or "I'm not sure I can cope with this."

Think how much worse it would be if you didn't have the Answer to cope with problems!

Recently Charles and I went to a conference where the main topic was survival. We've never heard so much gloom and doom in our entire lives. Charles and I are looking forward to the best years of our lives, though we're older than we have ever been before! We're looking forward not just to surviving, but to living the abundant life Jesus promised.

Wherever you go, the Lord always provides opportunities to minister in His name.

One day a man came into our office to see about some concrete work we needed. He had never seen a miracle, but before he got out of there, he saw his own leg grow out in divine healing. He was already saved, but he went on to receive the baptism with the Holy Spirit, which he had been seeking for years.

He walked out a different person! Sometimes we think that we shouldn't talk about Jesus to people with whom we do business because we think they might not be interested or because we think "business is business." I personally believe Jesus is the best business to talk about, and that's why we discuss Him all the time.

When God planted a seed in you, He did not plant that seed to die. He planted that seed to grow in you.

You apparently have something inside of you that makes you want to heal the sick, or you would not be reading this book. God has dropped a seed into your heart, and you need to nurture that seed and get a vision of what God has called you to do. Ignore circumstances that might try to change your mind.

Step 3: Have Confidence in God

It's easy to have confidence in God, because nothing is impossible with God. We all know He can do anything. We know He can heal the sickest person; through God the most crippled person can be healed and walk perfectly. But do we believe God can use us? We need to have confidence in God *in* us.

In Matthew 17:14-20 we read:

And when they had come to the multitude, a man came to Him, kneeling down to Him and saying, "Lord, have mercy on my son, for he is an epileptic and suffers severely; for he often falls into the fire and often into the water. So I brought him to Your disciples, but they could not cure him."

Then Jesus answered and said, "O faithless and perverse generation, how long shall I be with you? How long shall I bear with you? Bring him here to Me." And Jesus rebuked the demon, and it came out of him; and the child was cured from that very hour.

Then the disciples came to Jesus privately and said, "Why could we not cast it out?"

So Jesus said to them, "Because of your unbelief; for assuredly, I say to you, if you have faith as a mustard seed, you will say to this mountain, 'Move from here to there,' and it will move; and nothing will be impossible for you."

I want to burn the last part into your heart so that you will never forget it: "*And nothing will be impossible....*" If I stopped right there, it would be easy to agree with me. But if you read the entire clause, it says, "*And nothing will be impossible for you.*"

Jesus meant it. That is why He gave us the privilege of stepping out in faith and laying hands on the sick, knowing they will be healed. As you just read, He said that nothing will be impossible for you. He didn't say for *Me*, because we all know that nothing is impossible for Him. To think that nothing is impossible for us, however, certainly changes our way of thinking.

The apostle Paul wrote, "I can do all things through Christ who strengthens me" (Phil. 4:13). We need to get that in our spirits and know we cannot do it on our own, but that we can do all things — whatever God calls us to do — through Christ who strengthens us.

Often when I lay hands on people, I pause before I start and say: "I can do all things through Christ who strengthens me." Jesus made a positive statement in Mark 16: "Those who believe...will lay hands on the sick, and they will recover" (vv. 17-18). No *ifs, ands* or *buts* about it — "those who believe will lay hands on the sick, and they will recover."

John 14:12, one of my favoriteverses, says, "Most assuredly, I say to you, he who believes in Me, the works that I do he will do also; and greater works than these he will do, because I go to My Father."

I didn't say that — Jesus did! As a believer, I have the right, the privilege and the authority to do even greater things than He did. Not only that, I have a responsibility to fulfill the Word of God in me because God lives in me, and Jesus lives in and through me. We need to believe that God's Word is speaking directly and personally to us in this twentieth century.

Every time a new year rolls around, both Charles and I get excited because we anticipate all the great and wonderful things God is going to do through us. Then when we reach the middle of the year, we look back and say: "God, we're so grateful for what You did in the first six months. Now what are You going to do in the last six months?" He always tops what He did the first six months!

We all need to be reminded of our potential, because we often forget that we can do all things through Christ who strengthens us. I can do greater things than Jesus did, not because I say it, but because He says it in His Word!

When you have confidence in God in *you*, then you will realize you don't have to answer every voice of criticism. When you get in the healing ministry, people will criticize you. But we need to understand that taking criticism is a part of anyone's life who is on the front lines. So instead of confidence in the critical things that someone may have said to you, you need to have confidence in God in you.

Step 4: Be Persistent

If you want to be successful in healing, you must be persistent. You cannot let go the first time somebody comes up to you and says: "Who do you think you are to lay hands on the sick?"

That can either crush you or inspire you to pray, "Thank You, Father, that Your Word says I can lay hands on the sick, and they will recover."

The primary reason that some people fizzle out after a healing class or explosion is because they fail to persist. Maybe on your first healing trip or mission you

51

came against a hard case. To God no case is harder than another; but to us some seem harder than others. So we may encounter two or three people whom we classify as impossible cases. We think, I had three people with severed spinal cords, and not one of them got healed! Don't get discouraged! Be persistent! Keep on going! One of the most persistent men in the Bible was Elisha. He got a vision of what he wanted, and hung on — and he got exactly what he wanted (see 2 Kings 2).

Charles and I have often failed to see people healed. We have prayed for cancer victims who have died. But we have also prayed for many who lived. We keep right on going regardless of what happens, constantly learning more about healing in Jesus' name than we knew ten or fifteen years ago — or even one year ago. We are two of the most persistent people on earth.

Many people are healed when they quote, "By His stripes I am healed." It's wonderful when that happens. But there are times when someone leaves a healing service looking just as bad as when he or she arrived.

I often laugh at Charles. He will call to the stage someone who has a back problem. Sometimes he does what we normally do, and the person doesn't get healed right away. If something doesn't work, Charles tries another prayer or command. He is persistent, and I have almost never seen someone with a back problem fail to be healed.

You can give up easily and say, "Well, it isn't working." Yes, it is, because in the final analysis, it will!

If you want to be a successful Christian — one who is alive to the Holy Spirit all the time — you must be persistent in every area of your life: in reading the Bible; in winning people to Jesus; in talking about Jesus. All of these things are vital.

Be persistent! Don't give up! The devil is the one who comes in and says, "It's not going to work." If you've ever laid hands on someone, you've more than likely had a visit from the devil before you ever took your hands off! He'll tell you that your Christianity won't work. But the Bible tells us that we're victorious in all things and more than conquerors. I constantly say that everything I put my hand to prospers. Because I belong to Christ Jesus I am blessed with every spiritual blessing. Therefore it pleases God for me to walk in divine health.

You, too, need to be persistent in speaking the Word of God over yourself. Be persistent; don't give up. No matter how many times the devil comes against you, don't you ever give up. No matter how many times you think you have failed, hang in there. Be persistent.

Step 5: Know What You Are Doing

You can be ignorant but sincere, and God will honor that. It will help tremendously, however, if you learn everything you can about healing. I often am amazed at some of the things I did when I first got saved.

For instance, at the first church in which I ever spoke, I gave an altar call and didn't know what to do when people responded. I don't think I believed anyone would answer the altar call, so when the first person came, I thought to myself, What am I going to do with the people who come up?

When others came and began to tell me their requests, I was dumbfounded. Finally I said, "As soon as I get home, I'll start praying." Isn't it wonderful that God will bless us in spite of our ignorance? But I discovered that if I was going to speak in churches, I needed to learn how to minister to people at the altar, to meet their needs right there and to introduce them to Jesus — the One who can give them the answer to every problem they might have.

Likewise, learn as much as you possibly can about healing. You can't learn too much. Charles and I are constantly learning new things about healing. The other night we were watching some videotapes of old healing services. Many were from the crusades of men such as A. A. Allen and William Branham, who were well-known years ago for their tremendous healings on the "Voice of Healing" program. We watched a couple of hours of the actual live services they conducted, and we learned tremendous things from these men. Whenever we watch a healing service on television or go to someone else's healing service, we watch carefully to see if we can learn something new.

We love to watch the new "babies" at a healing explosion. Sometimes they do things they never learned but apparently were instructed to do by the Holy Spirit. We see them doing things we never thought about doing or saying, and we discover that what they do is effective.

Learn everything you can about healing from successful people. Don't learn things from individuals who never have any successes in their healing attempts. Receive instruction from those who have had successful experiences and who know what they're doing!

Although Charles and I wrote the book *How to Heal the Sick*, we still read it over and over because we forget some of the things we wrote. We watch the videotapes over and over, laughingly amazed at the fresh inspiration we receive from them each time. And every time I watch them, the Holy Spirit reminds me of something I have forgotten. When you watch those videos or read the book time and again, you'll learn something new every time.

Read the four Gospels and the book of Acts repeatedly to learn more about healing in the first-century church. I still read those five books more than any others because they talk about healing more than any other part of the Bible. If you want to learn how to heal, do the same things Jesus did. Say the same things Jesus said. You will be amazed at how effective that will be.

Two things bring miracles, and they go together — the name of Jesus and the power of God's Holy Spirit. The power Jesus displayed in His miracles came from His Father and from the Holy Spirit. Jesus said, "For the works which the Father has given Me to finish — the very works that I do — bear witness...that the Father has sent me" (John 5:36).

You also will be able to do miracles by using the name of Jesus and the power of God's Holy Spirit. Practice on everyone you can. Practice on your friends. Practice on your family and on yourself until you learn how to be proficient. The more you lay hands on the sick, the more proficient you'll become and the greater results you'll see.

Keep yourself prayed up! And keep yourself "read up" in the Bible at all times.

Step 6: Talk About Your Successes, Not Your Failures

When Charles and I write or speak, we always talk about success. We never tell about the people who don't get healed — we tell about the ones who do. In doing this, we have discovered that the more we talk about success, the more people get healed. As we tell the victory stories, everyone's faith rises.

I recently heard about a lady brought to one of our healing explosions on a stretcher, dying of cancer. The doctors had allowed her to come because they said she had less than twenty-four hours to live. This was more than a year ago, and we just heard that she was completely healed by the power of God. Now she's telling everyone what Jesus did to her when she came to a healing explosion.

Those are the kinds of stories to tell — the success stories. One of my favorite Scripture verses is Philippians 4:8: "Finally, brethren, whatever things are true, whatever things are noble, whatever things are just, whatever things are pure, whatever things are lovely, whatever things are of good report, if there is any virtue and if there is anything praiseworthy — meditate on these things."

Think about the good things; think about the praiseworthy things. Think about that crippled person who got out of a wheelchair; think about that person with the horrible back problem who got healed when her legs grew out! Don't tell people about your failures — tell them about your successes!

Step 7: Get to Know Him

If you want to have success in ministering healing biblically, get to know Jesus in the power of His resurrection.

Psalm 27:1-4 in the Living Bible is tremendous. There is a real clue in here.

> The Lord is my light and my salvation; whom shall I fear? When evil men come to destroy me, they will stumble and fall! Yes, though a mighty army marches against me, my heart shall know no fear! I am confident that God will save me .
>
> The one thing I want from God, the thing I seek most of all, is the privilege of meditating in his Temple, living in his presence every day of my life, delighting in his incomparable perfections and glory.

I don't know what part of that verse spoke to you the most clearly. But one day during a prayer meeting in our office, we asked the staff which part of that passage ministered to them the most.

One man said, "I am the most grateful for my salvation."

Another one said, "I just praise the Lord that He will protect me. Although an army marches against me, I will be protected."

Charles and I were thrilled the most by the part that says, "The thing I seek the most of all is the privilege of meditating in his Temple, living in his presence every day of my life."

When you get to know Jesus, you will have the same desires He has. The more you get to know Him, the closer you get to Him. The more intimate you become with Him, the more you will become like Him. The more you will have compassion in your heart to reach out to people who are lost, dying and sick.

The entire world desperately needs to know a living Jesus, but they also need you and me to introduce them to the One who is the answer to all of life's problems.

What an awesome privilege, yet what an equally awesome responsibility is given to us to bring the world to a living knowledge of the Lord Jesus Christ!

> But what things were gain to me, these I have counted loss for Christ. Yet indeed I also count all things loss for the excellence of the knowledge of Christ Jesus my Lord, for whom I have suffered the loss of all things, and count them as rubbish, that I may gain Christ and be found *in* Him, not having my own righteousness, which is from the law, but that which is through faith in Christ, the righteousness which is from God by faith; that *I may know Him* and the power of His resurrection (Phil. 3:7-10, italics added).

Verses 12 through 14 expound on other great things:

> Not that I have already attained, or am already perfected; but I press on, that I may lay

hold of that for which Christ Jesus has also laid hold of me. Brethren, I do not count myself to have apprehended; but one thing I do, forgetting those things which are behind and reaching forward to those things which are ahead, I press toward the goal for the prize of the upward call of God in Christ Jesus."

"I press toward the goal." Probably Paul's greatest desire was to *know* Him. To know Him more intimately than I can even dream possible is the desire of my heart.

The day I got saved I heard a song that said, "Turn your eyes upon Jesus, look full in His wonderful face. And the things of earth will grow strangely dim in the light of His glory and grace."[1]

The more you get to know Him, the dimmer the things of this earth will become and the less hold they will have on you. Put all of these seven steps into practice; think about them and meditate upon them. I guarantee they will lead you to success in ministering healing biblically.

Keep it up, remembering you are doing your part to usher in the King of kings and the Lord of lords.

And you are...
   well-equipped and
   dangerously loaded
   and
   have the ability to explode all over!

(Frances)

TEN

AS YOU
ARE GOING...

When Jesus told us to go, He meant "as you are going"— going about your daily business, at work, in school, at the park, at the shopping center, before and after church, in the restaurant, at the health club, at prayer meetings, at coffee or lunch breaks or wherever your daily life takes you. We should be fulfilling the Great Commission on a continual daily basis.

Walk, run or fly with us through a few of the life-style events of our normal daily walk with Jesus!

Flying to a meeting one day, the man sitting next to us stood up. We noticed a special back pillow in his seat. To us that was a signal for a miracle. When he returned, we questioned him about his back.

He was a salesman who traveled overseas as well as in the United States. He said the pain was so excruciating that he didn't believe he would be able to make it to Ireland the next week.

As we were getting off the plane in the next city, we asked him, "Would you like to go to the lobby and let us pray for your back to be healed?" When you're hurting badly enough, you will never resist such an offer. We told him he had nothing to lose.

He was in such severe pain as he hobbled to the lobby that he was almost in tears. He didn't want to sit down in public, so we put him behind the ticket counter wall. His back was so out of line, we discovered, that one leg was two inches shorter than the other leg. When it grew out, he jumped up, bent over, twisted his back and then heard, "Final boarding call!" He ran down the ramp as fast as he could, yelling, "I have no more pain!"

Another healing occurred when we stopped at a restaurant on a trip. After seating us at a dirty, oil-cloth-covered table, the waitress gave us the menus. Charles noticed something. He said to the waitress: "My wife has a wonderful ministry for pregnant women. Would you like for her to pray for you?"

The young woman burst into laughter and said, "Pray?" and continued laughing.

I immediately sensed a wonderful "as we were going" opportunity. So, grabbing her left hand, I laid my hand on her tummy and said: "Father, I thank You for this beautiful baby. Thank You that we don't believe in abortion." Before I said another word, she burst into tears. I knew she had considered abortion. I asked her whether she was married because there was no ring on her finger. She stumbled for words and finally came out with a very weak yes.

I said: "You need Jesus, honey. Pray this prayer after me."

She prayed, and when we finished, I asked her, "Where is Jesus right now?"

She said, "In my heart!" The girl we left behind was not the same girl we met when we came in. She was a new creature!

At a restaurant recently, a friend complained that her back was hurting. Charles immediately jumped up, measured her legs and commanded the back to be adjusted. She was instantly relieved of pain! Then he finished his dinner.

Don't get discouraged if you don't see an instant miracle. Some miracles happen the moment you lay hands on the sick — but other healings take time. Tell the person to whom you are ministering that the healing has started once you have laid hands on them. Do everything you can to keep people from becoming discouraged. Build their faith — and yours — with every sentence you speak.

We do not lay hands on the sick when we *feel* like it. We lay hands on the sick at every opportunity! Some of the greatest healings we have ever seen have taken place when we were sick or completely exhausted. Don't wait for a feeling — *do it now!*

When God opens a door for you, go through it. He always has something special for you on the other side. If an opportunity to lay hands on someone occurs — go for it — regardless of whether you *feel* anything or not. You'll be in the miracle ministry, too!

CHRISTIAN LIFE BOOKS
TOOLS FOR SPIRIT-LED LIVING

If you enjoyed *Healing*, we would like
to recommend the following books:

Effective Prayer
by John Dawson, B. J. Willhite, Francis MacNutt,
Judson Cornwall and Larry Lea

The Gifts of the Spirit
by Jack Hayford, John Wimber, Reinhard Bonnke,
Judith MacNutt, Michael P. Williams, Mark A. Pearson,
John Archer and Mahesh Chavda

Miracles Never Cease!
by William DeArteaga, Paul Thigpen, Jack Deere and Oral Roberts

Prophecy in the Church
by Martin Scott

God's Remedy for Rejection
by Derek Prince

Parents and Teachers: Equipping the Younger Saints
by David Walters

Living in the Supernatural
by Kathie Walters

God's Amazing Grace
by Terry Virgo

Available at your local Christian bookstore or from:

Creation House
190 North Westmonte Drive
Altamonte Springs, FL 32714
1-800-451-4598

Books by

Charles ❤ Frances Hunter

A Confession a Day Keeps the Devil Away
Angels on Assignment
Are You Tired?
Born Again! What Do You Mean?
Come Alive
Don't Limit God
Follow Me
Go, Man, Go
God Is Fabulous
God's Answer to Fat...Loøse It!
God's Conditions for Prosperity
Handbook for Healing
Hang Loose With Jesus
Healing — A Life-Style
His Power Through You
Hot Line to Heaven
How Do You Treat My Son Jesus?
How to Heal the Sick
How to Make Your Marriage Exciting
How to Overcome "Cool-Down" and Keep the Fire Burning
How to Receive and Maintain a Healing
How to Receive and Minister the Baptism
With the Holy Spirit
How to Win Your City to Jesus
I Don't Follow Signs and Wonders...They Follow Me!
If You Really Love Me...
Impossible Miracles
Memorizing Made Easy
My Love Affair With Charles
Nuggets of Truth
Possessing the Mind of Christ
P.T.L.A. (Praise the Lord, Anyway!)
Since Jesus Passed By
Strength for Today
Supernatural Horizons (From Glory to Glory)